MW01493615

Dr. Barl
for Diabetes

The Ultimate Guide on Treating
and Curing Diabetes with Natural
Barbara O'Neill Recommended
Herbs and Foods

ISBN 978-1-300-60035-0
Theodore Jamieson
Copyright@2025

TABLE OF CONTENT

CHAPTER 1

Introduction

Comprehensive Analysis of Diabetes (Type 1 and Type 2)

Diabetes mellitus, often known as diabetes, is a long-term medical condition marked by elevated levels of glucose (sugar) in the bloodstream. The body may either fail to produce sufficient insulin, a hormone responsible for regulating blood sugar levels, or may not utilize the insulin it does produce effectively. Diabetes is categorized into two primary types: Type 1 and Type 2.

Type 1 Diabetes: Also referred to as insulin-dependent diabetes or juvenile-onset diabetes, Type 1 diabetes is an autoimmune condition characterized by the immune system's attack on and destruction of the insulin-producing beta cells in the pancreas. This leads to minimal or absent insulin production. Individuals diagnosed with Type 1 diabetes necessitate continuous insulin therapy to effectively regulate their blood glucose levels. This form of diabetes generally manifests in children, adolescents, or young adults, although it can arise at any age. The symptoms of

Type 1 diabetes encompass frequent urination, excessive thirst, extreme hunger, unintended weight loss, fatigue, and blurred vision.

Type 2 Diabetes: Type 2 diabetes, often referred to as non-insulin-dependent diabetes or adult-onset diabetes, is a medical condition characterized by the body's resistance to insulin or insufficient insulin production by the pancreas, leading to abnormal blood sugar levels. This form of diabetes is prevalent and is frequently linked to factors such as advanced age, obesity, lack of physical activity, and a familial predisposition to diabetes. In contrast to Type 1 diabetes, Type 2 diabetes is frequently manageable through lifestyle modifications, including dietary adjustments and physical activity. In certain instances, medication or insulin therapy may also be necessary. The symptoms associated with Type 2 diabetes encompass heightened thirst, frequent urination, increased appetite, weight loss, fatigue, blurred vision, slow-healing sores, and a tendency for frequent infections.
Significance of Regulating Blood Sugar Levels

Effective management of blood sugar levels is essential for individuals with diabetes to avert complications and uphold overall health and well-being. Consistently elevated blood sugar levels can result in a variety of significant health complications, such as cardiovascular disease, nerve damage (neuropathy), kidney damage (nephropathy), eye damage (retinopathy), foot issues, skin conditions, and a heightened risk of infections.

Effective management of blood sugar entails a systematic approach that includes monitoring glucose levels, adhering to a nutritious diet, participating in consistent physical activity, and utilizing prescribed medications or insulin as necessary. Managing blood sugar levels is crucial for several important reasons:

Effective blood sugar management is essential in minimizing the risk of both immediate and long-term complications related to diabetes. Short-term complications encompass hypoglycemia (low blood sugar) and hyperglycemia (high blood sugar), both of which can pose serious risks if not addressed in a timely manner. Long-term complications, including heart disease, stroke, kidney failure, and vision loss, can greatly affect quality of life and result in disability or premature death.

Improving Quality of Life: Keeping blood sugar levels stable can assist individuals with diabetes in feeling better on a daily basis. Symptoms including fatigue, frequent urination, and excessive thirst can be effectively managed, enabling individuals to engage in a more active and fulfilling lifestyle.

Enhancing Energy Levels: Maintaining stable blood sugar levels can lead to improved energy levels and contribute positively to overall physical and mental well-being. Variations in blood sugar levels may result in fatigue, irritability, and challenges with concentration.

Facilitating Effective Weight Management: A balanced diet and consistent physical activity, essential elements of blood sugar regulation, can assist individuals in achieving and sustaining a healthy weight. Obesity represents a considerable risk factor for Type 2 diabetes, and reducing excess weight can enhance insulin sensitivity and blood sugar regulation.

Managing blood sugar levels effectively can help prevent the expensive complications associated with diabetes, thereby decreasing the necessity for medical interventions, hospitalizations, and medications.

CHAPTER 2

Understanding Diabetes

Factors and Considerations

Diabetes is a multifaceted metabolic condition marked by increased blood glucose levels, which can be influenced by a range of factors. The causes and risk factors for Type 1 and Type 2 diabetes are notably distinct.

Type 1 Diabetes:

Genetic Factors: Type 1 diabetes is significantly influenced by genetic elements. Those with a familial background of Type 1 diabetes face an increased likelihood of developing the condition. Specific genes linked to the immune system, including the HLA (human leukocyte antigen) genes, contribute to heightened susceptibility to Type 1 diabetes.

Type 1 diabetes is characterized as an autoimmune condition where the immune system erroneously targets and eliminates the insulin-producing beta cells located in the pancreas. The precise cause of this autoimmune response remains unclear; however, it is thought to result from a combination of genetic predisposition and environmental influences.

Environmental Factors: Although the precise environmental triggers remain unclear, elements such as viral infections (e.g., enteroviruses), early exposure to cow's milk, and other unidentified environmental agents may play a role in the onset of Type 1 diabetes.

Type 2 Diabetes:

Genetic factors significantly influence the development of Type 2 diabetes. Those with a familial background of Type 2 diabetes face a heightened risk of developing the condition. A number of genes linked to insulin resistance and beta-cell dysfunction have been identified.

Obesity and Physical Inactivity: Abdominal obesity is a significant risk factor for the development of Type 2 diabetes. Excess body fat, especially in the abdominal area, can result in insulin resistance, causing the body's cells to become less responsive to insulin. Physical inactivity worsens this condition by diminishing the body's capacity to utilize insulin effectively.

A diet characterized by elevated levels of refined sugars, unhealthy fats, and processed foods may play a significant role in the onset of Type 2 diabetes. The consumption of sugary beverages, fast food, and high-calorie snacks may contribute to weight gain and elevate the risk of insulin resistance.

The likelihood of developing Type 2 diabetes escalates as one ages. Although it can manifest at any age, its prevalence is higher among adults aged 45 and older.

Ethnicity: Specific ethnic groups, such as African Americans, Hispanic/Latino Americans, Native Americans, Asian Americans, and Pacific Islanders, exhibit an increased risk of developing Type 2 diabetes.

Medical Conditions: Conditions including polycystic ovary syndrome (PCOS), hypertension (high blood pressure), and dyslipidemia (abnormal lipid levels) are linked to a heightened risk of Type 2 diabetes.

Clinical Presentation and Assessment

Symptoms of Diabetes: The manifestations of diabetes may differ based on the specific type and the severity of the condition. The following are frequently observed symptoms:

Frequent urination, also known as polyuria, occurs when elevated blood sugar levels prompt the kidneys to filter out excess glucose from the bloodstream, resulting in increased urine production and the need to urinate more often.

Excessive thirst, known as polydipsia, occurs due to frequent urination, which results in dehydration and subsequently prompts an increase in thirst and fluid consumption.

Increased Hunger (Polyphagia): Individuals with diabetes may experience heightened hunger despite adequate food intake, stemming from the body's inefficiency in utilizing glucose for energy.

Unintended Weight Loss: In Type 1 diabetes, the body's lack of insulin production causes the breakdown of muscle and fat for energy, leading to unexplained weight loss.

Fatigue: Elevated blood sugar levels can lead to fatigue and weakness, as the body's cells lack the necessary glucose for energy production.

Blurred Vision: Increased blood sugar levels may result in fluid being drawn from the lenses of the eyes, which can lead to blurred vision.

Slow-healing sores can occur due to poor blood circulation and a diminished immune response in individuals with diabetes, leading to prolonged wound healing and an increased risk of infections.

Tingling or Numbness: Nerve damage resulting from elevated blood sugar levels may cause sensations of tingling, numbness, or discomfort in the hands and feet.

Diagnosis of Diabetes: The diagnosis of diabetes involves an assessment of medical history, a physical examination, and the utilization of laboratory tests. The primary diagnostic tests consist of:

The Fasting Plasma Glucose Test assesses blood glucose levels following a minimum fasting period of 8 hours. A fasting blood glucose level of 126 mg/dL (7.0 mmol/L) or greater on two distinct occasions signifies the presence of diabetes.

The Oral Glucose Tolerance Test (OGTT) assesses blood glucose levels prior to and following the intake of a glucose-rich beverage. Blood glucose levels are assessed at consistent intervals throughout a 2-hour duration. A blood glucose level of 200 mg/dL (11.1 mmol/L) or higher, measured 2 hours after eating, is indicative of diabetes.

The Hemoglobin A1c (HbA1c) test assesses the average blood glucose levels over the preceding 2 to 3 months. An HbA1c level of 6.5% or greater signifies the presence of diabetes.

The Random Plasma Glucose Test assesses blood glucose levels at any time throughout the day, independent of the individual's last meal. A random blood glucose level of 200 mg/dL (11.1 mmol/L) or higher, in conjunction with symptoms of diabetes, signifies the presence of the condition.

Complications Associated with Uncontrolled Diabetes

Unmanaged diabetes may result in various severe and potentially life-threatening complications. These complications may impact multiple organs and systems within the body:

Cardiovascular Disease: Diabetes notably elevates the risk of cardiovascular diseases, such as coronary artery disease, heart attack, stroke, and peripheral artery disease. Elevated blood sugar levels can harm blood vessels and lead to the accumulation of fatty deposits (atherosclerosis) within the arteries.

Diabetic neuropathy refers to nerve damage resulting from sustained elevated blood sugar levels. This condition may result in numbness, tingling, pain, and a loss of sensation, especially in the extremities, such as the hands and feet. Significant nerve damage may lead to complications such as ulcers, infections, and potentially necessitate amputation.

Diabetic nephropathy refers to kidney damage resulting from elevated blood sugar levels. It may result in compromised kidney function and ultimately lead to kidney failure. Diabetes ranks among the primary contributors to end-stage renal disease (ESRD), necessitating dialysis or kidney transplantation.

Diabetic retinopathy refers to the damage inflicted on the blood vessels within the retina, which is the light-sensitive tissue located at the rear of the eye, as a result of elevated blood sugar levels. It may result in vision complications, such as blurred vision, floaters, and potential blindness. Diabetes ranks among the primary contributors to adult blindness.

Foot Issues: Diabetes may result in inadequate blood circulation and nerve damage in the feet, which can lead to foot ulcers, infections, and delayed wound healing. In critical situations, amputation may be necessary to halt the progression of infection.

Skin Conditions: Individuals with diabetes exhibit an increased vulnerability to skin infections, fungal infections, and various skin conditions, including diabetic dermopathy and acanthosis nigricans.

Gastroparesis is a condition that can arise from diabetes, as the disease may impact the nerves responsible for stomach function, resulting in delayed gastric emptying. The symptoms presented are nausea, vomiting, bloating, and abdominal pain.

Elevated blood sugar levels can compromise the immune system, resulting in a higher susceptibility to infections for individuals with diabetes, such as urinary tract infections, respiratory infections, and skin infections.

CHAPTER 3

Natural Remedies for Managing Diabetes

Herbs and Supplements

For centuries, traditional medicine has utilized a range of herbs and natural supplements to assist in the management of blood sugar levels. Although these remedies should not serve as a substitute for conventional treatment, they can enhance a diabetes management plan when implemented with expert guidance. Below are several herbs and supplements recognized for their potential advantages in diabetes management:

Bitter Melon (Momordica charantia):

Bitter melon, referred to as bitter gourd, is a tropical fruit frequently utilized in traditional medicine due to its anti-diabetic properties. The fruit includes compounds such as charantin, vicine, and polypeptide-p, which have demonstrated blood glucose-lowering effects.

Advantages:

Bitter melon has been shown to enhance insulin sensitivity and facilitate glucose uptake by cells, contributing to the reduction of blood sugar levels.

Enhanced Glycemic Regulation: Certain studies indicate that bitter melon may lower HbA1c levels, which serve as an indicator of long-term blood glucose management.

Bitter melon can be utilized in multiple ways, such as fresh, in juice form, or as a dietary supplement. Consulting with a healthcare provider prior to using bitter melon is crucial, as it may interact with specific medications and has the potential to induce hypoglycemia (low blood sugar).

Fenugreek (Trigonella foenum-graecum):

Fenugreek is a herb frequently utilized in both culinary and medicinal applications. The seeds are rich in soluble fiber and contain compounds such as 4-hydroxyisoleucine, which have demonstrated anti-diabetic properties.

Advantages:

Enhanced Insulin Sensitivity: Fenugreek seeds have demonstrated the ability to improve insulin sensitivity and glucose tolerance.

The soluble fiber present in fenugreek seeds contributes to a gradual digestion and absorption of carbohydrates, leading to more stable blood sugar levels.

Fenugreek seeds may be soaked in water overnight and taken on an empty stomach, or incorporated into meals. Fenugreek supplements are readily accessible. Prior to using any supplement, it is essential to seek guidance from a healthcare professional.

Cinnamon (Cinnamomum spp.)

Cinnamon is a widely recognized spice known for its potential anti-diabetic properties. This product includes bioactive compounds such as cinnamaldehyde and polyphenols, which have the potential to enhance blood sugar regulation.

Advantages:

Cinnamon has demonstrated the ability to enhance insulin sensitivity, enabling cells to utilize glucose more efficiently.

Reduced Blood Sugar Levels: Certain studies indicate that cinnamon may assist in lowering fasting blood glucose levels and enhancing overall glycemic control.

Cinnamon can be incorporated into various foods and beverages, including oatmeal, smoothies, and tea. Cinnamon supplements are readily available. It is essential to recognize that high intake of cinnamon, particularly cassia cinnamon, may result in negative effects owing to its coumarin content. Ceylon cinnamon, characterized by its lower coumarin content, presents a more secure alternative.

Berberine:

Berberine is a bioactive compound present in various plants, such as goldenseal, barberry, and Oregon grape. This substance has been utilized in traditional Chinese and Ayurvedic medicine for its numerous health benefits, including its possible anti-diabetic properties.

Advantages:

Enhanced Insulin Sensitivity: Berberine has been shown to activate an enzyme known as AMP-activated protein kinase (AMPK), which is involved in metabolic regulation and the improvement of insulin sensitivity.

Blood Sugar Regulation: Research indicates that berberine may assist in reducing fasting blood glucose levels and enhancing HbA1c levels.

Berberine supplements are offered in both capsule and tablet forms. Adhering to the recommended dosage and seeking guidance from a healthcare professional is essential, as berberine may interact with specific medications and lead to gastrointestinal side effects.

Aloe Vera (Aloe barbadensis miller):

Aloe vera is a succulent plant recognized for its therapeutic benefits. The gel derived from its leaves comprises bioactive compounds such as polysaccharides and anthraquinones, which may exhibit anti-diabetic properties.

Advantages:

Enhanced Glycemic Regulation: Certain studies indicate that aloe vera gel may assist in reducing fasting blood glucose levels and improving HbA1c levels.

Aloe vera has the potential to enhance insulin sensitivity and facilitate glucose uptake by cells.

Aloe vera gel may be utilized as a dietary supplement or incorporated into beverages such as smoothies and juices. Utilizing products that are explicitly designated for internal use is crucial, and it is advisable to seek guidance from a healthcare provider prior to usage, as aloe vera may lead to gastrointestinal discomfort in certain individuals.

CHAPTER 4

Healthy Foods for Diabetes Management

Low Glycemic Index Foods

Whole Grains (Quinoa, Oats):

Whole grains serve as a valuable source of complex carbohydrates, fiber, vitamins, and minerals. Whole grains, in contrast to refined grains, possess a lower glycemic index, resulting in a more gradual increase in blood sugar levels.

Quinoa:

Nutritional Profile: Quinoa serves as a complete protein, offering all nine essential amino acids. It contains significant amounts of fiber, magnesium, iron, and antioxidants.

The advantages of quinoa in diabetes management include its high fiber content, which aids in slowing the digestion and absorption of carbohydrates, resulting in a gradual rise in blood sugar levels. The protein content contributes to increased satiety and aids in reducing overall calorie consumption.

Incorporating Quinoa: Quinoa is a versatile ingredient that can be utilized in a range of dishes, including salads, soups, and grain bowls. This option serves as a nutritious substitute for rice or pasta.

Oats:

Nutritional Profile: Oats contain a high level of soluble fiber, especially beta-glucan, which has demonstrated positive effects on blood sugar regulation. These products also include essential vitamins, minerals, and antioxidants.

The soluble fiber found in oats contributes to diabetes management by slowing the digestion and absorption of carbohydrates, resulting in more stable blood sugar levels. Oats have demonstrated the ability to enhance insulin sensitivity and lower the risk of cardiovascular disease.

Incorporating Oats: Oats serve as an excellent breakfast choice, including options like oatmeal or overnight oats. These can also be incorporated into smoothies, baked goods, and used as a coating for proteins such as chicken or fish.

Legumes (Beans, Lentils):

Legumes, such as beans and lentils, are highly nutritious foods that offer complex carbohydrates, fiber, protein, vitamins, and minerals. These foods possess a low glycemic index and serve as a valuable component of a diet suitable for individuals with diabetes.

Beans:

The nutritional profile of beans includes high levels of fiber, protein, folate, iron, and potassium. Various types of beans encompass black beans, kidney beans, chickpeas, and navy beans.

The high fiber content in beans aids in slowing the digestion and absorption of carbohydrates, resulting in more stable blood sugar levels for effective diabetes management. Beans serve as an excellent source of plant-based protein, contributing to feelings of fullness and aiding in weight management.

Beans can be integrated into salads, soups, stews, and chili. They can also be blended into spreads, such as hummus, or utilized as a meat alternative in various dishes.

Lentils:

The nutritional profile of lentils includes a high content of fiber, protein, folate, iron, and potassium. Lentils are available in several varieties, such as brown, green, red, and black.

Lentils offer advantages for diabetes management due to their low glycemic index and high fiber content, which contribute to the stabilization of blood sugar levels. They serve as an excellent source of plant-based protein and essential nutrients.

Lentils can be utilized in a variety of dishes, including soups, stews, salads, and curries. They may also be prepared and mashed to create spreads or utilized as a foundation for vegetable burgers.

Non-Starchy Vegetables (Broccoli, Spinach):

Non-starchy vegetables are characterized by their low carbohydrate and calorie content, positioning them as a highly suitable option for diabetes management. They are abundant in vitamins, minerals, fiber, and antioxidants.

Broccoli:

Broccoli is a cruciferous vegetable that boasts a rich nutritional profile, including vitamins C, K, and A, along with fiber, folate, and antioxidants like sulforaphane.

The advantages of managing diabetes include broccoli's significant fiber content, which aids in slowing the digestion and absorption of carbohydrates, resulting in more stable blood sugar levels. The presence of sulforaphane in broccoli demonstrates anti-inflammatory and antioxidant properties, potentially contributing to overall health and lowering the risk of complications related to diabetes.

Incorporating Broccoli: Broccoli may be prepared by steaming, roasting, sautéing, or consuming raw in salads. This ingredient can be incorporated into soups, stir-fries, and casseroles.

Spinach:

Spinach is a leafy green vegetable that boasts a rich nutritional profile, containing significant amounts of vitamins A, C, and K, along with folate, iron, calcium, and fiber.

Advantages for Diabetes Management: Spinach is low in carbohydrates and calories, positioning it as an ideal option for regulating blood sugar levels. The elevated nutrient content contributes to overall health and may assist in mitigating the risk of complications related to diabetes.

Incorporating Spinach: Spinach can be utilized in salads, blended into smoothies, or prepared in a variety of dishes including omelets, soups, and stir-fries. This product serves as an excellent base for pasta dishes and can also be incorporated into sandwiches and wraps.

Further Recommendations for Integrating Low Glycemic Index Foods:

Balanced Meals: Strive to incorporate a combination of low glycemic index foods, lean proteins, and healthy fats in every meal. This combination may assist in stabilizing blood sugar levels and delivering sustained energy throughout the day.

Portion Control: Although low glycemic index foods contribute positively to blood sugar management, it is crucial to implement portion control to prevent excessive calorie consumption. Careful monitoring of portion sizes can assist in maintaining a healthy weight and preventing fluctuations in blood sugar levels.

Meal Planning: Strategically plan meals and snacks in advance to guarantee the inclusion of a diverse range of low glycemic index foods in your diet. This approach can assist you in making healthier choices and in steering clear of high glycemic index or processed foods.

Maintaining a Consistent Eating Schedule: Consuming meals at regular intervals throughout the day can contribute to stable blood sugar levels. Strive to consume three well-balanced meals along with healthy snacks as necessary to maintain stable blood glucose levels.

Maintaining proper hydration is crucial for overall health and can aid in the management of blood sugar levels. Ensure adequate hydration by consuming ample water throughout the day while minimizing the intake of sugary beverages.

When shopping for packaged foods, it is essential to read labels to identify whole grain options and to avoid products that contain added sugars and refined carbohydrates. Seek out products that are designated as 100% whole grain and review the ingredient list for any concealed sugars.

Integrating low glycemic index foods like whole grains (quinoa, oats), legumes (beans, lentils), and non-starchy vegetables (broccoli, spinach) into your diet can be crucial for effective diabetes management. These foods offer vital nutrients, fiber, and protein, contributing to the stabilization of blood sugar levels.

Healthy Fats and Proteins
Nuts and Seeds

Nuts and seeds are highly nutritious foods that offer a rich source of healthy fats, protein, fiber, vitamins, and minerals. These foods possess a low glycemic index and can serve as a beneficial component of a diet suitable for individuals with diabetes.

Nuts:

The nutritional profile of nuts, including almonds, walnuts, pistachios, and pecans, reveals their richness in monounsaturated and polyunsaturated fats, protein, fiber, and essential nutrients such as vitamin E, magnesium, and potassium.

The healthy fats in nuts contribute to enhanced insulin sensitivity and a reduction in inflammation, which are beneficial for diabetes management. Their elevated fiber content moderates the digestion and absorption of carbohydrates, resulting in more consistent blood sugar levels. Nuts have been demonstrated to promote heart health, a crucial factor for individuals with diabetes who face a heightened risk of cardiovascular disease.

Nuts can be consumed as a snack, incorporated into salads, yogurt, or oatmeal, and utilized in cooking and baking. Selecting unsalted and raw or dry-roasted varieties is crucial to prevent the inclusion of added sodium and unhealthy fats.

Seeds:

The nutritional profile of seeds, including chia seeds, flaxseeds, pumpkin seeds, and sunflower seeds, reveals their richness in healthy fats, protein, fiber, and essential nutrients such as omega-3 fatty acids, antioxidants, and minerals.

Advantages for Diabetes Management: Seeds offer a source of healthy fats that may aid in reducing inflammation and enhancing insulin sensitivity. The fiber present in seeds contributes to the gradual digestion of carbohydrates and aids in maintaining stable blood sugar levels. Omega-3 fatty acids found in seeds such as flaxseeds and chia seeds demonstrate anti-inflammatory and heart-protective properties.

Incorporating seeds can enhance various dishes, including yogurt, smoothies, salads, and oatmeal. These can also be incorporated into baked goods, homemade granola, and energy bars. Ground flaxseeds and chia seeds serve as effective egg substitutes in baking.

Fatty Fish such as Salmon and Mackerel

Fatty fish serve as outstanding sources of omega-3 fatty acids, high-quality protein, vitamins, and minerals. Omega-3 fatty acids are vital fats recognized for their various health advantages, especially concerning cardiovascular health and inflammation management.

Salmon:

The nutritional profile of salmon includes a significant amount of omega-3 fatty acids (EPA and DHA), high-quality protein, as well as vitamins B12 and D, along with essential minerals like selenium and potassium.

The inclusion of omega-3 fatty acids found in salmon offers significant advantages for diabetes management, as they possess anti-inflammatory properties and may enhance insulin sensitivity. They contribute to cardiovascular health by decreasing triglyceride levels, lowering blood pressure, and inhibiting the formation of blood clots. The protein found in salmon offers sustained energy and supports the maintenance of muscle mass.

Incorporating Salmon: Salmon may be prepared through grilling, baking, broiling, or poaching methods. This item can be incorporated into salads, sandwiches, or served as a main dish. Smoked salmon can be incorporated into whole-grain crackers, salads, or utilized in omelets and frittatas.

Mackerel:

Nutritional Profile: Mackerel is a fatty fish that is abundant in omega-3 fatty acids (EPA and DHA), high-quality protein, vitamins B12 and D, as well as essential minerals like selenium and phosphorus.

Benefits for Diabetes Management: Like salmon, mackerel offers anti-inflammatory omega-3 fatty acids that may enhance insulin sensitivity and promote heart health. The protein content contributes to the stabilization of blood sugar levels and the preservation of muscle mass.

Mackerel can be prepared through grilling, baking, or broiling methods. This item can serve as a main dish, be incorporated into salads, or be utilized in spreads and pâtés. Canned mackerel serves as a practical choice for preparing swift and uncomplicated meals.

Lean Proteins and Plant-Based Sources

Protein is a vital nutrient that contributes to the building and repairing of tissues, the production of enzymes and hormones, and the maintenance of overall health. Incorporating lean meats and plant-based proteins into a diabetes-friendly diet can deliver essential protein while minimizing saturated fats.

Lean Meats:

The nutritional profile of lean meats, including chicken, turkey, and lean cuts of beef and pork, offers high-quality protein along with essential vitamins, such as B vitamins, and important minerals like iron and zinc.

Advantages for Diabetes Management: Lean meats contain lower levels of saturated fats in comparison to fattier cuts, presenting a healthier choice for individuals with diabetes who face a heightened risk of cardiovascular disease. Protein derived from lean meats contributes to the stabilization of blood sugar levels and the preservation of muscle mass.

Incorporating lean meats can be achieved through grilling, baking, broiling, or roasting methods. They may serve as a main dish, be incorporated into salads, or be utilized in wraps and sandwiches. Avoiding breaded and fried meats is essential, as they can contribute unhealthy fats and carbohydrates to your diet.

Plant-Based Proteins:

The nutritional profile of plant-based proteins, including beans, lentils, tofu, tempeh, and edamame, offers high-quality protein, fiber, vitamins, and minerals. They are also minimal in saturated fats and cholesterol.

Advantages for Diabetes Management: Plant-based proteins provide a heart-healthy substitute for animal proteins. Their elevated fiber content contributes to the stabilization of blood sugar levels and enhances insulin sensitivity. Research indicates that plant-based diets are linked to a reduced risk of developing Type 2 diabetes and improved glycemic control.

Incorporating plant-based proteins such as beans and lentils can enhance soups, stews, salads, and chili. Tofu and tempeh are versatile ingredients suitable for incorporation into stir-fries, curries, and sandwiches. Edamame serves as a versatile option, suitable for snacking or enhancing salads and grain bowls.

Further Recommendations for Integrating Healthy Fats and Proteins:

Balanced Meals: Strive to incorporate a combination of healthy fats, lean proteins, and low glycemic index carbohydrates in every meal. This combination may assist in stabilizing blood sugar levels and delivering sustained energy throughout the day.

Implement portion control to prevent excessive calorie consumption. Although healthy fats and proteins offer advantages, excessive consumption can result in weight gain.

Incorporate a diverse selection of healthy fats and proteins into your diet to guarantee a comprehensive intake of essential nutrients. Incorporate a variety of nuts, seeds, fatty fish, lean meats, and plant-based proteins into your diet.

Utilize healthy cooking techniques including grilling, baking, broiling, steaming, and roasting to prepare your meals. Refrain from deep-frying and utilizing excessive amounts of oil and butter.

When shopping for packaged foods, it is essential to read labels to identify products that contain healthy fats and proteins. Refrain from selecting products that contain added sugars, unhealthy fats, and high levels of sodium.

Including healthy fats and proteins like nuts and seeds, fatty fish such as salmon and mackerel, as well as lean meats and plant-based proteins in your diet can be crucial for effective diabetes management. These foods offer vital nutrients, promote cardiovascular health, and assist in maintaining stable blood sugar levels.

Fruits and Their Impact on Blood Sugar
Blueberries and Strawberries

Berries are strongly advised for individuals with diabetes because of their low glycemic index and significant nutritional benefits.

Blueberries:

The nutritional profile of blueberries includes a rich array of vitamins C and K, fiber, and powerful antioxidants like anthocyanins.

Advantages for Blood Sugar Regulation: Blueberries have demonstrated the ability to enhance insulin sensitivity and reduce blood sugar levels. The elevated fiber content contributes to a slower digestion and absorption of sugars, resulting in a more gradual increase in blood glucose levels. The antioxidants found in blueberries contribute to reducing inflammation and offer protection against oxidative stress, thereby enhancing overall health.

Incorporating Blueberries: Blueberries may be consumed fresh or frozen, integrated into yogurt, oatmeal, smoothies, and salads, or utilized in various baking recipes. They serve as a delightful and healthful snack independently.

Strawberries:

The nutritional profile of strawberries includes high levels of vitamin C, manganese, folate, and fiber. These also include antioxidants such as anthocyanins and ellagic acid.

The fiber and antioxidants present in strawberries contribute to the regulation of blood sugar levels and the reduction of inflammation. Their low glycemic index guarantees a minimal effect on blood glucose levels. Furthermore, strawberries have the potential to enhance cardiovascular health by reducing cholesterol levels.

Incorporating Strawberries: Strawberries may be enjoyed fresh or frozen, included in cereals, yogurt, salads, and smoothies, or utilized in nutritious desserts. They offer versatility and can elevate both sweet and savory dishes.

Apples and Pears

Apples and pears are commendable options for individuals managing diabetes, as they offer high fiber content and a low glycemic index.

Apples:

The nutritional profile of apples includes a high content of dietary fiber, especially pectin, along with significant amounts of vitamins C and A, and a variety of antioxidants.

The soluble fiber in apples effectively slows the digestion and absorption of carbohydrates, leading to a gradual increase in blood sugar levels. Apples are rich in polyphenols, which have demonstrated the ability to enhance insulin sensitivity and lower the risk of cardiovascular disease. Consuming apples with the skin intact offers enhanced fiber and nutrient content.

Incorporating Apples: Apples can be consumed fresh, sliced with nut butter, included in salads, or utilized in cooking and baking. They can also be prepared as applesauce without added sugars, providing a nutritious snack alternative.

Pears:

The nutritional profile of pears includes a high content of fiber, vitamin C, and potassium. These also include antioxidants like flavonoids.

The high fiber content in pears contributes to the stabilization of blood sugar levels by slowing the absorption of sugars. Pears possess a high water content, contributing to overall hydration and promoting a sense of fullness.

Pears can be consumed fresh, incorporated into salads, or utilized in various cooking and baking applications. Much like apples, retaining the skin enhances fiber content and nutrient availability. Pears may also be poached to create a delightful and nutritious dessert.

Citrus Fruits (Oranges, Grapefruits)

Citrus fruits are recognized for their significant vitamin C content and numerous health advantages. Although they contain natural sugars, these foods possess a low glycemic index and can be incorporated into a diet suitable for individuals with diabetes.

Oranges:

Nutritional Profile: Oranges are an excellent source of vitamin C, fiber, folate, and potassium. They also include flavonoids and various antioxidants.

The fiber content in oranges contributes to the regulation of blood sugar levels by slowing the digestion and absorption of sugars, resulting in a more gradual increase in blood sugar levels. The antioxidants present in oranges exhibit anti-inflammatory properties and contribute to overall health. It is advisable to consume whole oranges instead of orange juice to maximize the intake of fiber.

Incorporating Oranges: Oranges can be consumed fresh, included in salads, or utilized in smoothies. They may also complement savory dishes, enhancing the overall flavor profile. Orange segments provide a refreshing enhancement to a diverse range of meals.

Grapefruits:

The nutritional profile of grapefruits includes a high content of vitamin C, fiber, vitamin A, and antioxidants like lycopene.

The fiber content in grapefruits aids in the regulation of blood sugar levels by decelerating the absorption of sugars. The antioxidants found in grapefruits possess anti-inflammatory properties and contribute to cardiovascular health. Caution is advised regarding grapefruit consumption when taking specific medications, as grapefruit may interact with a range of drugs.

Incorporating Grapefruits: Grapefruits may be consumed fresh, included in salads, or utilized in smoothies. Grapefruit segments contribute a tangy flavor profile that enhances both sweet and savory dishes. Moderate consumption of grapefruits can yield health benefits while maintaining stable blood sugar levels.

Further Suggestions for Integrating Fruits into a Diabetes-Friendly Diet

Portion Control: Although fruits are nutritious, it is important to implement portion control to prevent excessive carbohydrate consumption. A standard serving size generally consists of one small piece of fruit, half of a large fruit, or a half-cup of either fresh or frozen fruit.

Combining fruits with a source of protein or healthy fats can assist in stabilizing blood sugar levels. For instance, consider pairing an apple with nut butter or incorporating berries into yogurt for a well-rounded snack option.

Whole fruits are more advantageous than fruit juices, as they provide fiber that aids in regulating blood sugar levels. Fruit juices may lead to quick increases in blood glucose levels and do not contain the advantageous fiber present in whole fruits.

Regularly Monitor Blood Sugar Levels: It is essential for individuals with diabetes to consistently monitor their blood sugar levels to comprehend the impact of various fruits on their glucose levels. This can assist in making informed dietary decisions.

Incorporate a diverse selection of fruits into your diet to guarantee a comprehensive intake of nutrients. Incorporate a variety of fruits into your diet to take advantage of their distinct health benefits.

Integrating fruits like berries (blueberries, strawberries), apples, pears, and citrus fruits (oranges, grapefruits) into your diet may be advantageous for diabetes management. These fruits offer vital vitamins, minerals, fiber, and antioxidants, and they possess a low glycemic index, rendering them appropriate for managing blood sugar levels.

CHAPTER 5

Lifestyle Tips for Diabetes Management

Regular Physical Activity
Advantages of Physical Activity:

Enhanced Regulation of Blood Glucose Levels:

Engaging in exercise facilitates the utilization of glucose by muscles for energy, thereby contributing to a reduction in blood sugar levels. Engaging in physical activity enhances insulin sensitivity, enabling the body to utilize insulin more efficiently. The outcomes may result in improved glycemic control and diminished blood glucose variability.

Weight Management:

Consistent physical activity contributes to both weight loss and the maintenance of a healthy weight. Maintaining a healthy weight is essential for effectively managing Type 2 diabetes, as excess body fat, especially in the abdominal area, is linked to insulin resistance.

Cardiovascular Health:

Engaging in exercise enhances heart function and promotes better circulation, thereby lowering the risk of cardiovascular conditions including heart attack, stroke, and hypertension. This holds particular significance for individuals with diabetes, as they face an elevated risk of cardiovascular complications.

Enhanced Mental Well-being:

Engaging in physical activity stimulates the release of endorphins, which serve as the body's natural mood enhancers. Engaging in regular exercise can effectively alleviate stress, anxiety, and depression, thereby enhancing mental health and overall well-being.

Improved Muscle Strength and Flexibility:

Engaging in exercise contributes to the development and preservation of muscle mass, increases strength, and promotes flexibility. This approach can assist in injury prevention, enhance balance, and facilitate daily activities.

Improved Rest:

Engaging in regular physical activity can enhance sleep quality and duration, which is essential for overall health and effective diabetes management. Inadequate sleep can adversely affect blood sugar levels and insulin sensitivity.

Categories of Appropriate Exercises:

Strolling:

Advantages:

Walking is an uncomplicated, low-impact form of exercise that is available to the majority of individuals. This activity necessitates no specialized equipment and can be performed in a variety of locations. Walking contributes to the reduction of blood sugar levels, enhances cardiovascular health, and aids in weight management.

Methods for Integration:

Strive to engage in a minimum of 30 minutes of brisk walking on the majority of days each week. This can be divided into shorter sessions, such as three 10-minute walks. Integrate walking into your daily routines by considering options such as commuting on foot, utilizing stairs instead of elevators, or taking a stroll following meals.

Yoga:

Advantages:

Yoga integrates physical postures, breathing techniques, and meditation practices. This practice enhances flexibility, strength, and balance, while also fostering relaxation and alleviating stress. Research indicates that yoga can enhance insulin sensitivity and improve blood sugar regulation.

Methods for Integration:

Engage in a yoga class or utilize online videos designed specifically for beginners. Strive to engage in yoga for a minimum of 30 minutes multiple times each week. Concentrate on gentle, restorative yoga techniques that prioritize relaxation and stress alleviation.

Strength Training:

Advantages:

Strength training, often referred to as resistance training, encompasses exercises designed to develop and sustain muscle mass. It enhances insulin sensitivity, boosts metabolic rate, and aids in weight management. Strength training enhances bone density and lowers the risk of osteoporosis.

Methods for Integration:

Utilize free weights, resistance bands, or bodyweight exercises to conduct strength training routines. Strive to incorporate a minimum of two non-consecutive days of strength training weekly, focusing on all major muscle groups. Begin with lighter weights and progressively elevate the intensity as strength develops.

Supplementary Categories of Exercises:

Aerobic Exercises:

Activities include swimming, cycling, dancing, and aerobics classes.

Aerobic exercises contribute to improved cardiovascular fitness, assist in weight management, and enhance insulin sensitivity. They assist in reducing blood pressure and cholesterol levels.

To incorporate exercise effectively, strive for a minimum of 150 minutes of moderate-intensity aerobic activity or 75 minutes of vigorous-intensity aerobic activity each week. Select pursuits that you find enjoyable and can maintain over an extended period.

Exercises for Flexibility and Balance:

Examples include tai chi, Pilates, and stretching exercises.

The advantages of flexibility and balance exercises include improved joint mobility, a decreased risk of falls, and enhanced overall physical function. These exercises may provide significant advantages for older adults managing diabetes.

To incorporate these exercises effectively, aim to include flexibility and balance activities in your routine a minimum of two to three times per week. Concentrate on stretching all primary muscle groups and engaging in activities that enhance balance.

Interval Training:

Examples include high-intensity interval training (HIIT) and low-intensity interval training (LIIT).

Interval training involves alternating between brief periods of high-intensity activity and intervals of rest or lower-intensity exercise. It has the potential to enhance cardiovascular fitness, elevate calorie expenditure, and improve insulin sensitivity.

To incorporate interval training into your routine, alternate between high-intensity and low-intensity exercises. For instance, vary your routine by alternating between sprinting and walking or cycling at different intensity levels. Begin with shorter intervals and progressively extend both the duration and intensity.

Guidelines for Safe Exercise:

Engage with Healthcare Professionals:

Prior to initiating any new exercise regimen, it is essential to seek guidance from healthcare professionals, particularly if you have any pre-existing medical conditions or complications associated with diabetes. They are capable of delivering tailored recommendations and guaranteeing that the exercise plan is both safe and effective.

Regularly assess blood glucose levels:

Monitor blood sugar levels prior to, during, and following exercise to gain insights into how physical activity influences your glucose levels. This approach can assist in preventing hypoglycemia (low blood sugar) or hyperglycemia (high blood sugar) and facilitate necessary adjustments to your exercise regimen.

Maintain Adequate Hydration:

Ensure adequate hydration by consuming sufficient water before, during, and after exercise. Dehydration can impact blood sugar levels and overall performance.

Utilize Appropriate Footwear:

Select shoes that are comfortable and well-fitted, ensuring they offer sufficient support and cushioning. This holds particular significance for individuals with diabetes who may face an increased risk of foot complications. Regularly inspect your feet for any indications of injury or irritation.

Begin at a moderate pace and progressively elevate the intensity.

Start with low-intensity exercises and progressively enhance both the duration and intensity as your fitness level advances. This approach can assist in minimizing injuries and enhancing the overall experience of exercise.

Pay Attention to Your Body:

Observe your body's reactions to exercise carefully. Should you encounter any pain, dizziness, or atypical symptoms, please cease the activity and seek advice from a healthcare professional. Prioritizing safety and well-being is essential.

Stress Management
Significance of Stress Reduction

Effectively managing stress is essential for successful diabetes management. Chronic stress can adversely impact both physical and mental health, especially for those living with diabetes. Here are the reasons why minimizing stress is essential:

Effects on Blood Glucose Levels:

The release of stress hormones, including cortisol and adrenaline, is triggered by stress, leading to an increase in blood sugar levels. In individuals with diabetes, this may result in hyperglycemia (high blood sugar) and complicate the maintenance of stable glucose levels.

Insulin Resistance:

Chronic stress may lead to insulin resistance, a condition characterized by the body's cells becoming less responsive to insulin. This may worsen Type 2 diabetes and complicate blood sugar management.

Unhealthy Coping Strategies:

Stress may result in detrimental coping mechanisms, including overeating, the intake of sugary foods, smoking, or excessive alcohol consumption. The aforementioned behaviors may adversely affect blood sugar regulation and overall health outcomes.

Mental Health:

Chronic stress may lead to mental health challenges, including anxiety and depression. The relationship between mental health and diabetes management is significant, as individuals experiencing mental health challenges may encounter difficulties in following treatment plans and adopting healthy lifestyle choices.

Quality of Sleep:

Stress can negatively impact both the quality and duration of sleep, resulting in inadequate rest. Insufficient sleep can interfere with blood sugar regulation and insulin sensitivity, thereby complicating the management of diabetes.

Immune Function:

Chronic stress has the potential to compromise the immune system, resulting in increased vulnerability to infections and illnesses. This situation raises significant concerns for individuals with diabetes, who face an elevated risk for complications.

Methods for Alleviating Stress

Various effective methods exist for alleviating stress and encouraging relaxation. Integrating these practices into daily routines can assist individuals with diabetes in managing stress and enhancing their overall well-being. Here are several techniques to consider:

Meditation:

Advantages:

Meditation is a practice of mindfulness that entails concentrating one's attention and removing distracting thoughts. It facilitates relaxation, diminishes stress, and improves overall mental clarity. Consistent meditation practices can contribute to lowering blood pressure, alleviating anxiety, and enhancing emotional well-being.

Methods for Practicing:

Locate a serene and comfortable area to either sit or recline. Shut your eyes and concentrate on your breathing, paying attention to the feeling of each inhalation and exhalation. Should your thoughts drift, kindly redirect your attention to your breathing. Begin with a few minutes each day and progressively extend the duration as you gain more confidence in the practice. Numerous forms of meditation exist, including guided meditation, loving-kindness meditation, and body scan meditation, allowing you to explore and identify what suits you best.

Deep Breathing:

Advantages:

Deep breathing exercises facilitate the activation of the body's relaxation response, thereby diminishing stress and fostering a sense of tranquility. Deep breathing has the potential to decrease heart rate, alleviate muscle tension, and enhance oxygenation, thereby contributing to overall well-being.

Methods for Practicing:

Assume a comfortable seated or lying position. Position one hand on your chest and the other on your abdomen. Inhale slowly and deeply through your nose, permitting your abdomen to expand as you fill your lungs with air. Exhale gradually through your mouth, allowing your abdomen to descend. Continue this practice for several minutes, concentrating on the cadence of your breathing. Practicing techniques such as diaphragmatic breathing, box breathing, and 4-7-8 breathing can facilitate relaxation.

Interests:

Advantages:

Participating in hobbies and enjoyable activities can offer a mental respite from stressors while fostering a sense of fulfillment and relaxation. Engaging in hobbies can positively influence mood, alleviate anxiety, and contribute to an improved overall quality of life.

Suggestions for Hobbies:

Engaging in activities such as gardening, hiking, dancing, and sports offers significant physical and mental advantages.

Engaging in creative activities such as painting, drawing, writing, and crafting can serve as a therapeutic outlet and facilitate emotional expression.

Engaging in intellectual activities such as reading, solving puzzles, acquiring a new language, or playing musical instruments can enhance cognitive function and foster a sense of achievement.

Engaging in social activities such as spending time with friends and family, participating in clubs or groups, and volunteering can enhance social connections and provide support.

Further Strategies for Alleviating Stress:

Activity:

Engaging in physical activity serves as an effective means of alleviating stress. Engaging in exercise promotes the release of endorphins, which serve as natural enhancers of mood. Consistent exercise can enhance physical fitness, improve mental clarity, and alleviate stress and anxiety. Strive to engage in a minimum of 150 minutes of moderate-intensity aerobic exercise each week, in conjunction with strength training and flexibility exercises.

Mindfulness:

Mindfulness entails focusing on the current moment with an objective perspective. Engaging in mindfulness practices can lead to decreased stress levels, improved emotional management, and an overall enhancement of well-being. Mindfulness techniques encompass mindful breathing, mindful eating, and body scan meditation. Integrating mindfulness into everyday tasks, including eating, walking, or brushing your teeth, can enhance a sense of calm and awareness.

Effective Time Management:

Effective time management can alleviate stress by enabling individuals to prioritize tasks, establish realistic goals, and develop a balanced schedule. Implementing strategies like developing to-do lists, establishing deadlines, and dividing tasks into manageable steps can enhance productivity and alleviate feelings of being overwhelmed.

Community Assistance:

Establishing and nurturing robust social connections can offer emotional support and alleviate feelings of isolation. Engaging with loved ones, participating in support groups, and pursuing counseling can effectively manage stress and enhance mental well-being.

Methods for Relaxation:

Techniques such as progressive muscle relaxation, guided imagery, and aromatherapy are effective in promoting relaxation and alleviating stress. Progressive muscle relaxation entails the systematic tensing and subsequent relaxation of various muscle groups throughout the body, whereas guided imagery focuses on the visualization of serene and tranquil scenes. Aromatherapy employs essential oils to enhance relaxation and overall well-being.

Choices for a Healthy Lifestyle:

Adopting a healthy lifestyle can facilitate effective stress management. This encompasses maintaining a balanced diet, ensuring proper hydration, obtaining sufficient sleep, and limiting the intake of alcohol and caffeine. Adopting a healthy lifestyle can enhance both physical and mental resilience in the face of stress.

Developing a Stress Management Plan:

Recognize Stressors:

Identify the sources of stress in your life, including those associated with work, relationships, health, or other influences. Recognizing the factors that contribute to your stress can assist you in formulating effective strategies for its management and resolution.

Establish Achievable Objectives:

Establish realistic objectives for managing stress. Begin with small, manageable steps and progressively integrate additional techniques into your routine. Recognize your achievements and modify your strategy as necessary.

Establish a Routine:

Develop a daily schedule that incorporates time for activities aimed at reducing stress. Consistency is essential for maximizing the advantages of these practices. Engage in morning meditation, take lunchtime walks, or pursue evening hobbies to ensure you allocate time for activities that foster relaxation and well-being.

Seek assistance from qualified experts:

If stress becomes overwhelming or unmanageable, consider seeking assistance from a counselor, therapist, or healthcare provider. Support can offer valuable guidance and resources for managing stress.

Adequate Sleep and Its Role in Blood Sugar Control

The Significance of Sufficient Sleep

Hormonal Regulation:

Sleep plays a crucial role in regulating hormones that govern appetite and metabolism. Leptin and ghrelin are two essential hormones influenced by sleep. Leptin, known for its role in appetite suppression, diminishes with inadequate sleep, whereas ghrelin, which promotes appetite, rises in response. This imbalance may result in heightened hunger and excessive consumption, especially of high-calorie, sugary foods, which can adversely affect blood sugar levels.

Insulin Sensitivity:

Insulin sensitivity pertains to the efficiency with which the body's cells react to insulin. Proper sleep is essential for sustaining optimal insulin sensitivity, enabling cells to utilize glucose more effectively for energy production. Inadequate sleep can contribute to insulin resistance, causing cells to become less responsive to insulin, which leads to increased blood glucose levels.

Stress Hormones:

Sleep plays a crucial role in regulating stress hormones, including cortisol. Chronic sleep deprivation can result in elevated cortisol levels, which may lead to increased blood sugar levels by stimulating glucose production in the liver. Elevated cortisol levels may also play a role in the development of insulin resistance.

Inflammation:

Sufficient sleep contributes to the reduction of inflammation within the body. Chronic sleep deprivation is linked to elevated levels of inflammatory markers, which may lead to insulin resistance and the onset of Type 2 diabetes. Inflammation may further complicate issues related to diabetes.

Growth Hormone:

Sleep facilitates the secretion of growth hormone, which is essential for regulating metabolism and preserving muscle mass. Growth hormone facilitates glucose uptake by cells and contributes to overall metabolic health.

Mental Well-Being:

The relationship between sleep and mental health, as well as emotional well-being, is significant. Inadequate sleep may contribute to mood disorders, including anxiety and depression, which can adversely affect the management of diabetes. Mental health challenges can complicate adherence to treatment plans and the pursuit of healthy lifestyle choices.

The influence of sleep on blood sugar regulation

Blood Glucose Levels:

Proper sleep contributes to the stabilization of blood glucose levels by fostering hormonal balance and enhancing insulin sensitivity. Inadequate sleep can result in variations in blood sugar levels, complicating the effort to attain glycemic control. Individuals with diabetes experiencing sleep disturbances may observe elevated blood sugar levels upon waking (dawn phenomenon) or during the day.

Glycemic Variability:

Glycemic variability denotes the changes in blood glucose levels that occur over the course of the day. Elevated glycemic variability is linked to a higher risk of complications related to diabetes. Proper sleep contributes to minimizing glycemic variability by facilitating stable glucose regulation and enhancing insulin sensitivity.

Hypoglycemia:

Inadequate sleep may elevate the likelihood of nocturnal hypoglycemia (low blood sugar during the night) for individuals with diabetes who are utilizing insulin or specific medications. Nocturnal hypoglycemia may interfere with sleep patterns and result in fatigue and confusion upon awakening.

Nutrition Selections:

Insufficient sleep may result in suboptimal dietary decisions, including a higher intake of sugary and calorie-dense foods. These choices may result in fluctuations in blood sugar levels, complicating the management of diabetes.

Exercise:

Proper sleep enhances physical energy and motivation, facilitating regular participation in physical activity. Exercise plays a crucial role in managing blood sugar levels, while inadequate sleep can hinder the ability to sustain an active lifestyle.

Strategies for Enhancing Sleep Quality

Establish a regular sleep schedule:

Establish a consistent sleep schedule by going to bed and waking up at the same time each day, including weekends. Maintaining a consistent sleep schedule is essential for regulating the body's internal clock and enhancing sleep quality.

Establish a Calming Bedtime Routine:

Create a soothing pre-sleep routine to indicate to your body that it is time to relax. Engaging in activities like reading, enjoying a warm bath, practicing relaxation techniques, or listening to calming music can effectively facilitate your transition to sleep.

Establish an environment that promotes restful sleep.

Make certain that your sleep environment is comfortable and promotes restful sleep. Maintain a cool, dark, and quiet environment in the bedroom. Consider utilizing blackout curtains, earplugs, or white noise machines as necessary. Consider investing in a high-quality mattress and pillows for optimal comfort.

Minimize Screen Exposure:

Minimize the use of electronic devices, including smartphones, tablets, and computers, for at least one hour prior to bedtime. The blue light emitted by screens can disrupt melatonin production, a hormone essential for regulating sleep.

Be Mindful of Your Diet:

It is advisable to refrain from consuming heavy meals, caffeine, and alcohol in proximity to bedtime. These factors can interfere with sleep and influence blood sugar levels. If you find yourself hungry before bedtime, consider choosing a light, balanced snack.

Participate in Consistent Exercise:

Consistent physical activity can enhance sleep quality and aid in the regulation of blood sugar levels. It is advisable to refrain from engaging in vigorous physical activity near bedtime, as this may impede the ability to fall asleep.

Effectively Handle Stress:

Engage in stress-reducing techniques including meditation, deep breathing, or yoga. Minimizing stress can enhance sleep quality and support improved blood sugar regulation.

THE END

Made in United States
Troutdale, OR
06/10/2025

32030657R00040